THE HEAL
TRAUMA COMFREY

Terry Lemerond *and*
Holly Lucille, ND, RN

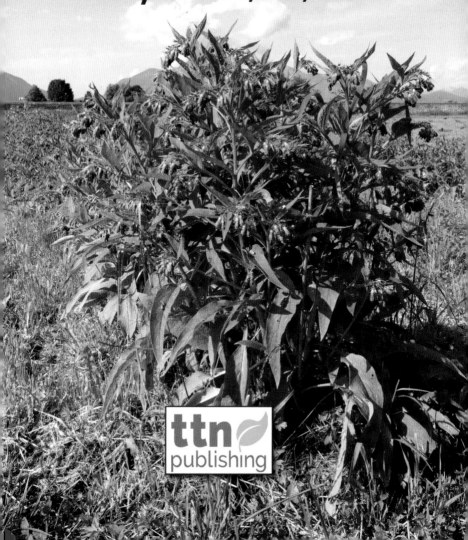

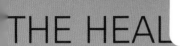

The purpose of this book is to educate. It is not intended to serve as a replacement for professional medical advice. Any use of the information in this book is at the reader's discretion. This book is sold with the understanding that neither the publisher nor the author has any liability or responsibility for any injury caused or alleged to be caused directly or indirectly by the information contained in this book. While every effort has been made to ensure its accuracy, the book's contents should not be construed as medical advice. To obtain medical advice on your individual health needs, please consult a qualified health care practitioner.

Copyright © 2021 Terry Talks Nutrition Books, Green Bay, WI

ISBN: 978-1-952507-14-4

Typesetting/graphic design: Gary A. Rosenberg • TheBookCouple.com
Editor: Kathleen Barnes

Printed in the United States of America

10   9   8   7   6   5   4   3   2   1

Contents

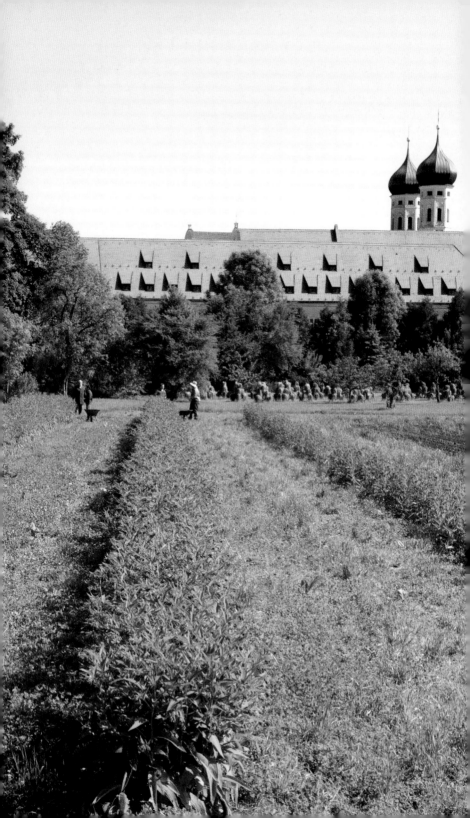

Introduction

I got my nickname, "Daredevil Doctor," after my episode on ABC's *Wipeout* aired early last year. You see, all my life I have had the need to hurl my body through space at daring speeds on either horses, motorcycles or just by itself. I also am an avid outdoors person and adore outback backpacking, gardening and playing just about any sport. Later in life, I found Crossfit, became certified as a coach and now I am a competitive athlete.

At my age, the game is all about staying safe, recovering well and keeping my skin in the game. That is why I absolutely love and depend on the healing powers of Trauma Comfrey. This powerful plant is with me everywhere I go. It is in my gym bag, my backpack, my book bag and even in my purse. I don't leave home without it.

—Holly Lucille, ND, RD

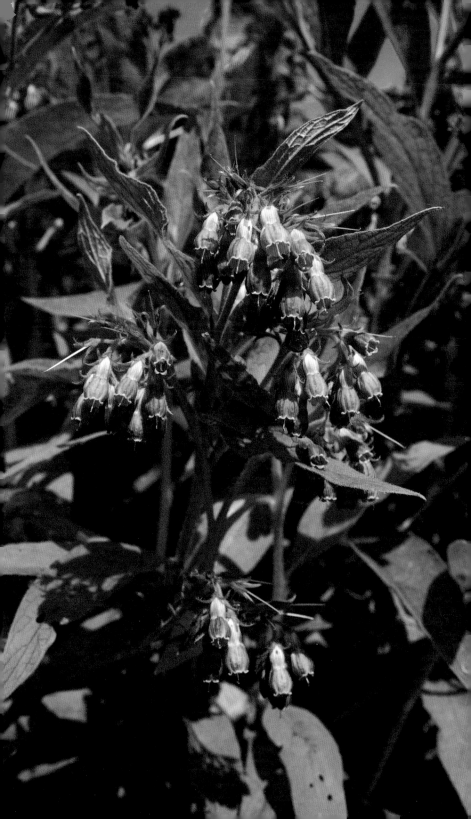

CHAPTER ONE

· · · · ·

What Is Comfrey?

If you've ever had a sprained ankle, a black-and-blue bruise or an aching back—and who hasn't?—then you know how much suffering these injuries can cause. Even though they're not life-threatening, they can make your days miserable with throbbing pain that seems to take forever to go away. Throughout the ages, we've endured the pain of these injuries unaware we could find quick relief with an amazingly potent herb that was close at hand: comfrey.

The story of comfrey is truly fascinating. Used by millions for millennia as medicine and food, it was largely forgotten in the last half-century, but a thrilling next chapter for this ancient herb is unfolding right now. Scientists have recently validated its healing effects, and they have learned how to amplify its curative properties with the latest agricultural and processing techniques. What's more, it has become easily and quickly available, even to modern city-dwellers far from a garden. That means that you don't have to fear being sidetracked by a simple injury ever again! That's the exciting news that we're going to share with you in the following pages.

Falls, blows, fractures, sprains, muscle aches, back and joint pain—these have always been part of the human experience. These days we're more likely to incur them on a tennis court than from behind a plow, and to treat them, we might get a splint at a doctor's office or grab a product off a pharmacy shelf. But way back when—as far back as 2,000 years ago—people would walk into a field or garden and reach for a plant with prickly leaves and purplish flowers. They called it by names like Knitback or Boneset, and it did exactly that—it knit broken skin and muscles and bones back together in record time.

Today, few people know of comfrey and even fewer would know what to do with it if handed a leaf or flower. They might complain that it's too prickly or too sticky. That's too bad, because with today's health challenges, we need every potent, natural healing agent we can find. And the latest groundbreaking research gives us even more reason to have comfrey by our side in a new, easily applied formulation perfect for our 21st century needs. But first, to appreciate its unique functions, let's dip into its colorful history:

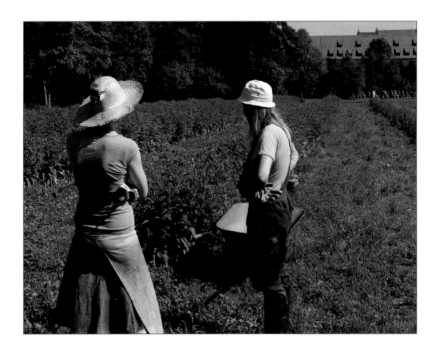

- If you were a wounded charioteer in ancient Rome, physicians would apply comfrey leaves on you to stop heavy bleeding.

- If you were a warrior in the armies of Alexander the Great that swept across Asia in the first century, you would get a comfrey poultice for a battle wound. Medics in armies from the U.S. Revolutionary War to World War I used comfrey as well.

- As a Cherokee in pre-European America, you would use comfrey—*oo ste e oo ste*—in sacred ceremonies, and you'd also drink it like tea to heal ulcers, purify blood, and get a good night's sleep. NOTE: Comfrey is now banned in the U.S. for internal use.

- In the Middle Ages in Europe, if you stumbled on rocks while chasing goats or injured your hand while laying a stone, monks at the local monastery would pick comfrey from their garden to treat your injury.

- If after giving birth, your breasts were sore from nursing, you applied a comfrey poultice.

For many hundreds of years, no *Materia Medica*—handbooks used by doctors of the time—was complete without detailed instructions on comfrey. Medical journals carried stories of near-miraculous healings. For example, a British nine-year-old named Samuel Thomson, who later became a leading botanical physician, severely injured his foot while using a piece of farm machinery. Amputation seemed the only option until comfrey poultices were applied to his foot and complete healing followed. In another case, the head of the Irish Royal College of Surgeons reported that after surgery failed for a man with a malignant tumor on his face, the man returned three months later completely cured—by applying comfrey poultices.

With the discovery of antibiotics in 1928, herbal medicine fell out of use in the United States and many parts of Europe, as doctors and patients turned to quick-acting drugs marketed as the latest innovations. It is only now, as we are starting to understand the limitations, expenses and side-effects of pharmaceuticals, that people in large numbers are re-examining the profound healing processes that natural herbs have to offer.

What exactly is comfrey?

Words are revealing, and when you look at this herb's many names, you can see what practical uses people have made of it.

The common name Comfrey stems from the Latin word *conferta,* meaning "to unite." Its official botanical name is *Symphytum officinale: Symphytum* means "to make grow together" and *officinale* refers to a monastery storeroom for botanical remedies, the pharmacy of its day. Its popular names also reveal its powers: Knitback, Bruisewort (wort meaning plant), Knitbone, Boneset.

Comfrey seems to have originated on the Asian steppes, in Eastern Europe and China and Russia. Easily propagated through its roots, it spread rapidly throughout Europe and Asia. Today it is found in temperate zones throughout the world, including the United States, sometimes growing wild near streams.

A perennial herb, comfrey belongs to the Boraginaceae family, which includes borage and forget-me-not. The plant is stout— about three feet high—and so thick that it's difficult to grow anything underneath it. Its root is brownish-black and the width of a turnip. To propagate it, even a tiny piece of the root will do. Its roots dive deep, as far as 12 feet down, enabling it to bring to the surface the rich minerals of the subsoil. Its dark green leaves are tapered like a lance, are hairy and bristly to the touch, and

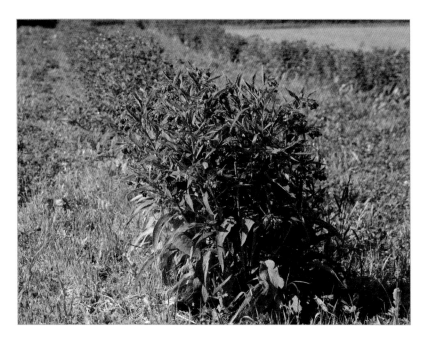

can grow to 18 inches in length. Its flowers are delicate and bell-shaped, and they can be white, blue, pink, or purple.

What makes comfrey so special?

Here's why comfrey is so powerful as a healer: It soothes pain, slows down further damage to tissues and fast-forwards the production of cartilage, tendons and muscles. It quickly and efficiently rebuilds damaged blood, bone and flesh. That's precisely what is needed for injuries including wounds, sores, burns, cuts, scrapes, bites, stings, rashes, swollen tissue, sprains and broken bones.

The most remarkable of comfrey's healing ingredients is called allantoin. It's known as a "cell proliferator" because it encourages cells to grow at a rapid rate—not in the chaotic manner of cancer cells, but in an orderly, orchestrated fashion as Nature intended.

This makes wounds heal faster. It is also enhances white blood cell production to help ward off many types of infections and diseases.

Actually, we've all had the allantoin experience—when our mothers were pregnant, a gland in the umbilical cord produced allantoin, thus helping the rapid cell growth in our embryonic bodies. A mother's milk after delivery is also rich in allantoin. So you might say that when our cells are bruised and battered from an injury, allantoin rushes to the rescue like a caring mother.

Allantoin, sometimes in its comfrey form, is used in many cosmetic products ranging from skin creams to shampoos and even toothpaste, because of its moisturizing effect and its ability to bond with and envelope irritating agents.

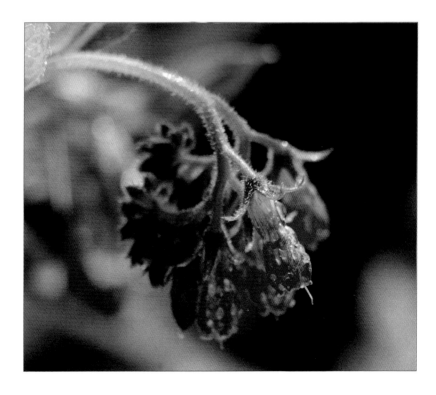

Another clue to comfrey's healing powers is the vibrant, dark green color of its leaves. That shows just how rich they are in chlorophyll, which scientists have found helps to rejuvenate old cells and accelerate the growth of new ones. Because its molecular structure resembles our blood, chlorophyll purifies blood, which speeds the healing process.

Comfrey also boasts a host of vitamins—strong doses of A, as well as B1, B2, B3, B5, B6, B12, C and E. It has 15 essential minerals, including calcium, phosphorus, potassium, chromium, cobalt, copper, magnesium, iron, manganese, sodium, boron, lead, sulphur, molybdenum, and zinc. Its constituents also include amounts of mucilage (a moist, sticky substance), pyrrolizidine (more on this compound in the next chapter), tannins (dark-colored compounds with a bitter taste), saponins (glucosides that form soapy lathers when mixed with water), asparagine (an amino acid), inulin (a soluble fiber), resins (sticky, flammable compounds), and phenolic acids including rosmarinic and caffeic, that protect cells from oxidative damage. Up to 35% of comfrey is protein, about as high a proportion as legumes, but it's not a good idea to eat it because some forms of comfrey have been associated with liver damage. (For more on completely non-toxic forms of comfrey, see Chapter 6.)

Although you might call allantoin the star player, all these components dance together in a complex choreograph of healing. They interact with each other biochemically in hundreds of ways we have yet to understand, and the effect is to provide a balanced interplay of nutrients to the body to maximize the healing process. It is this innate balance that makes herbs relatively safe compared to pharmaceuticals in which one component is removed from the rest, synthesized and pumped up to create specific results, usually with side effects.

Scientists have found that comfrey has an impressive array of healing properties:

Anti-bacterial	Kills or slows down growth of bacteria
Anti-exudative	Counters the oozing of fluid from cells and tissues as a result of inflammation or injury
Anti-fungal	Fights fungus invaders such as yeast, mold and rot
Anti-inflammatory	Prevents or reduces inflammation in cells
Anodyne	Relieves pain
Antiseptic	Kills or retards the growth of infection-causing microorganisms
Astringent	Draws tissue together, thus restricting the flow of blood
Alterative	Restores healthy functioning of the body
Demulcent	Soothes pain in inflamed tissues, especially mucous membranes
Emollient	Softens the skin
Expectorant	Helps the respiratory tract to expel phlegm and mucus
Homeostatic	Helps the body balance internal and external stress
Styptic	Arrests bleeding by contracting blood vessels
Tonic	Invigorates and restores health
Vulnerary	Heals fresh wounds
Pectoral	Relieves chest and respiratory disorders

How can you use comfrey?

In today's modern life, using the living comfrey plant is far from easy. First of all, there's the time and trouble involved. When you have a sprained ankle, you may not want to take to the time and effort to process it yourself: first of all, find a comfrey plant at just the right time in its growth cycle, then get purified water, then cut the plant's leaves and grind away at them with a mortar and pestle until you get a paste, then heat the mixture up to the right temperature, spread the sticky concoction over your ankle, wrap a bandage around it, and leave it on until it dries out—at which point you start the entire process over.

Furthermore, you need to have just the right kind of comfrey. If you use the Russian Comfrey found in British marshes and North American gardens, or the Prickly Comfrey or Quaker Comfrey often seen ornamentally, your efforts won't yield as potent a healing agent as your ankle deserves.

But not to worry! There is a much better option—a highly potent form of comfrey that you can simply squeeze from, yes, a tube! Let's explore just how this exciting development came about.

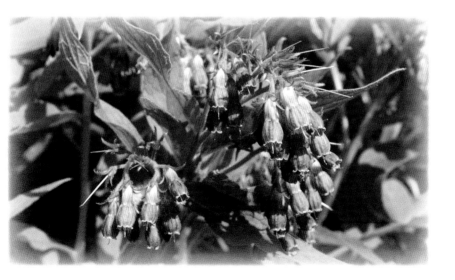

Fun Facts About Comfrey

- Travelers in the Middle Ages carried comfrey as a talisman to protect them and used it in magic spells to attract money.

- Comfrey roots have been used to dye clothes brown, to tan leather, and to spin Angora fleece.

- A healthy comfrey plant will live more than two decades.

- Comfrey is richer in nitrogen and phosphorus than many commercial fertilizers. It is used by many organic gardeners to fertilize crops, to break down foods in compost heaps, and as mulch.

- Early American settlers carried precious comfrey seeds with them from Europe—only to discover the plant already growing in their new land.

- In the 1800s, Europeans planted comfrey to attract bees, birds and butterflies to gardens. It was also widely used as fodder to make animals strong and resilient.

- Native Americans used comfrey leaves as pouches. When they folded a leaf, its small hairs stuck together like natural Velcro!

CHAPTER TWO

. . . . .

What Is
Trauma Comfrey?

In the foothills of the Bavarian Alps, on a gently rolling stretch of land that belongs to a Benedictine monastery, lies a very special garden. It holds rows upon rows of a particularly healing variety of comfrey. The crop is grown organically and gently: no pesticides, no herbicides, no chemical fertilizers touch these plants, only the fragrant breezes and gentle rains coming off the mountains. It is harvested by hand with scythes, not by machines. The result is what has become known as Trauma Comfrey, a plant as pure as that grown in the Middle Ages—and even more potent.

Those very plants, hung with purplish-pink trumpet flowers, are what make it possible to achieve fast wound healing right at home.

You see, as wonderful as comfrey is, not all varieties are created equal. As comfrey spread throughout the world, from Siberia to North Africa to North America and Australia, hybrids developed through cross-pollination by bees and through natural selection. Today, there are more than three dozen recognized varieties of Symphytum (comfrey) sold by commercial nurseries. Here are a few of the more popular varieties you'll see around:

- *Symphytum asperum* (Prickly Comfrey)

- *Symphytum grandiflorum* (Large-Flowered Comfrey)

- *Symphytum ibericum* (Dwarf Comfrey)

- *Symphytum officianale* (Common Comfrey)

- *Symphytum orientale* (White Comfrey)

- *Symphytum tuberosum* (Tuberous Comfrey)

Each of these has its particular mix of constituents. Among all these varieties, the one grown in the Bavarian Alps, *Symphytum x uplandicum* NYMAN is a bright star because it has particularly high levels of the following healing constituents:

- Allantoin, which stimulates the rebuilding of cells and regenerates damaged tissue in record time. It can actually travel through the skin all the way to tendons, cartilage and bone.

- Choline, an essential nutrient that kick-starts the recovery process, helps injured blood vessels and nerve endings to recover, and improves the pumping of healing blood through inflamed tissues.

- Rosmarinic acid, which fights inflammation, counters the oozing of fluid from cells and tissues as a result of injury, and slows down cell damage.

The unique nature of these particular plants has been protected by the European Plant Variety Office in a similar way to a patent. Its approved name? *Trauma Comfrey!*

For health-conscious, careful consumers like you, Trauma Comfrey has a critical advantage: its leaves, stems and flowers are completely free of a comfrey constituent called pyrrolizidine alkaloids, PAs for short. These are substances found also in pasture grasses like Ragwort and Heliotrope that, when ingested in high quantities over long periods of time, can cause liver disease, particularly in people with weak livers or who take liver-stressing medications. In two studies, some rats who were fed a diet extremely high in those ordinary forms of comfrey or who were injected with megadoses of a PA extract developed liver damage or tumors. Although comfrey has been used for many centuries as a food and a medicine, several countries (including the United States, Canada and Germany) decided to err on the side of safety and ban the use of comfrey in products designed for internal use and use on open wounds. However, Trauma Comfrey is totally safe to be applied to wounds because, unlike other forms, it is free of these toxic PA alkaloids.

For our own protection, it's important to know about PAs, but it's also important to know that when used externally, as salves or gels or poultices, safety in comfrey is not considered an issue because the skin does not easily absorb PAs. No country has restricted the external use of comfrey.

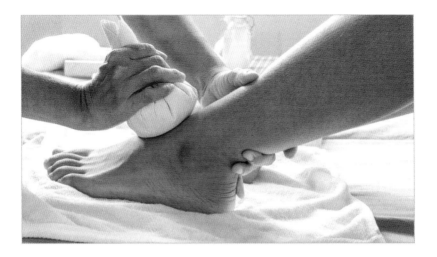

Trauma Comfrey is safe

Nevertheless, every step has been taken to make Trauma Comfrey products as safe as possible. First of all, Trauma Comfrey has been cultivated to contain undetectable amounts of PAs. The way in which it is harvested—using only the PA-free, nutrient-rich leaves, stems, and flowers rather than roots that typically have a higher PA content—adds another layer of protection. It is processed into a potent extract within hours after harvest by a laboratory that specializes in herbal preparations. The plants are continuously checked and double-checked to remove any stray PAs as well as to detect any contaminants such as toxic heavy metals or

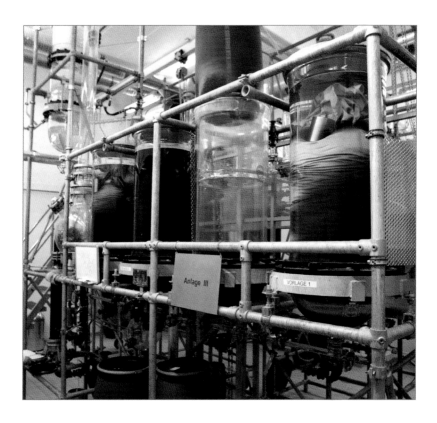

cancer-causing aflatoxins. By the time it gets to consumers, we can all rest assured that there are no harmful PAs, even though a cream made specifically from Trauma Comfrey should not be taken internally.

In a 2008 medical journal article, researchers reported that, when analyzed with the latest techniques and equipment—liquid chromatography electrospray ionization mass spectrometry—not even a trace of PAs was found in either the leaves and flowers of Trauma Comfrey or its extract.

That means that Trauma Comfrey delivers a powerful healing effect without any downsides!

Best of all, scientists at European institutes and universities have conducted so many studies on the topical application of Trauma Comfrey that its safety, tolerance and effectiveness have been repeatedly and resoundingly verified. They have found it to be so safe that it's approved for children over the age of four in Germany and approved for children over the age of two by Swiss authorities. It's found to be so effective that it can even ease the pain of chronic lower-back conditions. The coming chapters will help us look closely at that research to learn more about this amazing plant and product.

The Monastery Connection

The history of comfrey and monasteries have long been inter-twined. During the Middle Ages, monks were the physicians of their time and their herbal storerooms acted as the local pharmacies. It was a rough period of human history with perennial conflict and constant wars, and monastery gardens were full of comfrey because it was so effective at healing wounded soldiers and civilians. Even today, if you walk around the ruins of abandoned monasteries from Britain to the Caucasus, you'll often find comfrey growing out of the nooks and crannies between the stones!

The Benedictine monastery in which Trauma Comfrey is grown was founded in 739 A.D.—that means more than 1,200 years of continuous comfrey cultivation!

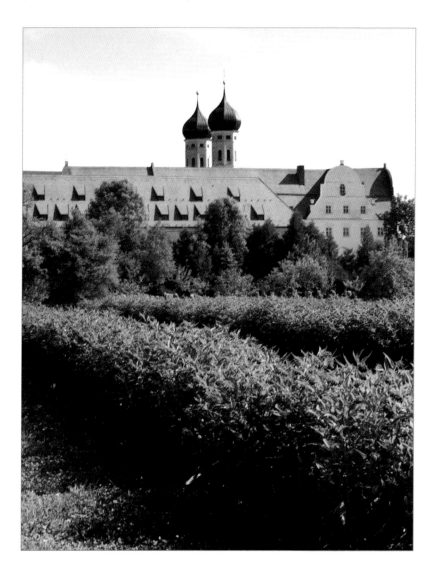

· · · · ·

CHAPTER THREE

Sports and Other Injuries: Healing Sprains, Strains, and Bruises

We Americans love to play and watch sports of all kinds, no doubt about it. But our national passion has a definite downside—injuries of all kinds. Just turn on a sports channel this weekend. Scarcely a football, basketball or hockey game ends without a muscular player lying flat on his back, moaning in pain. Or watch a football or soccer game on a playing field near your home: you don't have to be a player's mother to have your heart in your throat when a child or teen gets the wind, or worse, knocked out of them. For that matter, stop in at a fitness club or a yoga studio, and someone in a bandage might well limp past you.

Youthful sports injuries

Since the numbers of these types of injuries are rising, we adults look in the mirror and decide to get serious about exercise as increasing numbers of our children play competitive sports.

Sports injuries start young. According to the U.S. Centers for Disease Control, more than a third of all American children have suffered sports or recreational injuries that required treatment by a doctor or nurse. That comes to five million children a year!

No sport is free of risk for kids. The grade- and middle-school children who are injured include 28% of all football players, 25% of baseball players, 22% of soccer players, 15% of basketball players, and 12% of softball players. Injuries are suffered more often by girls before puberty, and by boys after puberty. A child is most likely to get injured in the early stages of learning a sport. The older the child, severe injury becomes more likely.

Children Ages 5 to 14 Treated in Emergency Rooms	
Bicycling	200,000
Basketball	170,000
Football	215,000
Baseball and softball	110,000
Trampolines	65,000
Soccer	88,000
Skateboarding	66,000
In-line and roller skating	47,000
Skiing/snowboarding	25,000
Gymnastics	23,500
Ice hockey	18,000
Sledding	15,000
Ice skating	10,600
TOTAL sports injuries treated in ERs:	775,000

—Source: Stanford Children's Health

Adults are vulnerable, too

Many of us adults—both those who are super-fit and "weekend warriors"—also have our share of hard knocks. Take runners— those thin, fit folks running through city parks at the break of dawn. Two-thirds of them are injured every year in a way that forces them to cut back their running time. Walkers? 21% injure themselves annually. What about badminton? A mild sport, right? Wrong—85 % of both elite and recreational players are injured in an average year!

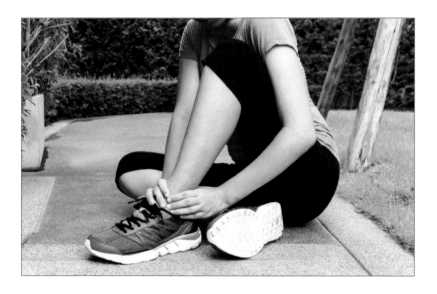

Some sports injuries come from impact with other players or their equipment and can't be easily avoided if you're playing hard. But in other sports, such as running, cycling, swimming and walking, the injuries most often come from "overuse." This means that you're straining your body beyond its capacity and it breaks down in some way. Injuries are more likely to happen if you're a newcomer to a sport rather than someone who's been training in it for many years. Worse yet, about half of all sports injuries are actually repeats of previous injuries!

Of course, sports aren't the only cause of injuries that range from inconvenient to life-changing. Car accidents, falls, blows from falling or hurtling objects can happen to anyone at any age. People stumble over rugs, fall off ladders, hit their thumbs with hammers and overexert themselves gardening or shoveling snow when they're at home.

And our jobs—especially physically demanding ones—take their toll. Among working people, 41% of all injuries in men and 33% of all injuries in women happen in the workplace, from activities like moving heavy supplies, tripping over wires or repetitive motion tasks.

And then there's the aging process itself. Although people over 65 increasingly pursue activities like bicycling and weight training, one in three older adults suffers a fall each year that can cause bruises and fractures; 2 to 30% suffer moderate to severe injuries such as lacerations, hip fractures or head traumas. The Centers for Disease Control and Prevention says 3 million older adults were treated in emergency rooms for falls and 800,000 of them are hospitalized. Once they are traumatized, many older people become fearful of activity, counterintuitively increasing their risk of injuries.

Types of injuries

Let's look more closely at the most common types of injuries, causes, and how Trauma Comfrey can make a big difference in recovery rates.

About 95% of sports injuries involve minor "soft tissue

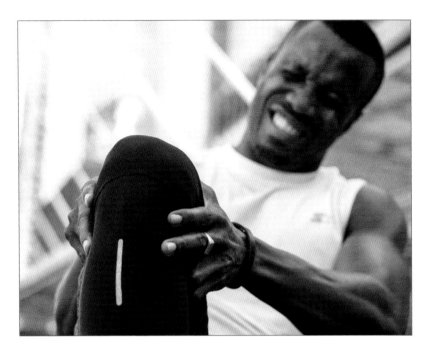

traumas" including muscles, ligaments and tendons, associated sprains, strains, tears, ruptures and bruises. They are known as "intact-skin" injuries because the skin is not broken. Another type of injury is "non-intact skin"—such as abrasions and wounds. We'll look at those in the next chapter.

Most of the intact-skin injuries are relatively minor in nature, which is not to say that they can't be extremely painful. They can affect movement and lifestyle in profound ways and may take months to completely heal. Let's look at some of them.

Sprains

Sprains are the result of stretching or tearing of the ligaments that connect the bone ends in joints. When you stress a joint, the ligament can overstretch or tear. You'll feel it immediately as a searing pain.

According to the Mayo Clinic, the most common places for sprains are:

- Ankle—Walking or exercising on an uneven surface

- Knee—Pivoting during an athletic activity

- Wrist—Landing on an outstretched hand during a fall

- Thumb—Skiing or playing racquet sports, such as tennis

Symptoms typically include pain, swelling, bruising and difficulty moving the joint.

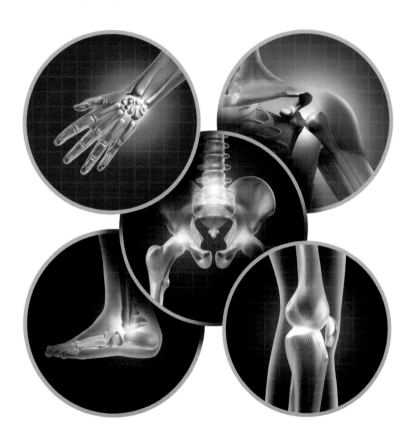

Strains

A strain occurs when you stretch, twist or tear a muscle or a tendon, the fibrous cord of tissue that connects muscles to bones. They commonly occur in the lower back and the hamstring muscle in the back of your thigh. The strain is labeled "acute" when a muscle stretches unusually far or abruptly. This could be the result of slipping on ice, running, jumping, throwing or lifting a heavy object. It is considered "chronic" if the strain results from prolonged, repetitive movement of a certain muscle, such as you might get by keyboarding, playing tennis, or rowing a boat. Typical symptoms are pain, swelling, muscle spasms, and difficulty moving the muscle.

Bruises

Called "contusions" in medical literature, bruises occur when blood vessels under the skin are broken and blood cells collect near the surface of the skin. A bruise can start out reddish, then will turn blue or dark purple in a few hours, and eventually fade to yellow or green before disappearing. They typically occur when we bump into something or when something bumps into us—what doctors call "blunt trauma"—and they can also result from over-exercise and blood thinning medications. The symptoms include pain and tenderness that usually recede as the color fades.

How these injuries are usually treated

Doctors have developed a simple four-step process for treating most of these injuries, which usually can be done at home as long as there is no broken bone, fever or open cut. It is known as the RICE method:

R—Rest the injured area, but don't avoid all activity.

I—Ice the area as soon as possible after the injury, ideally for 20 minutes every hour.

C—Compress the area by wrapping an elastic bandage around it.

E—Elevate the injured area above heart level to limit swelling.

If the pain is severe, doctors also recommend an over-the-counter NSAID (non-steroidal anti-inflammatory drug) such as ibuprofen, aspirin or acetaminophen. This, however, has its risks, since aspirin or ibuprofen slow down blood clotting and may prolong the bleeding. Acetaminophen is easy to overdose on because it is included in more than 500 medications; it causes half the cases of acute liver failure in the United States and is responsible for 26,000 hospitalizations and 500 deaths annually. (Contrast this with fewer than 12 reports of comfrey-related health problems

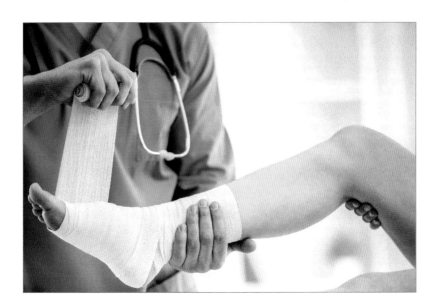

over several decades!) You may also require an oral pain relieving product, and rather than using an NSAID, curcumin is a natural anti-inflammatory that has been found to significantly reduce pain. Trauma Comfrey and curcumin, especially high absorption BCM-95 curcumin, would make an excellent combination for many forms of pain. For more information on the benefits of curcumin, we recommend Dr. Jan McBarron's book, *Curcumin, The 21st Century Cure.*

How Trauma Comfrey fast-forwards the healing process

As we've seen, comfrey—once called by such practical names *as Knitback, Boneset,* and *Bruisewort*—has unique healing attributes that made it the go-to remedy for injuries for 2,000 years. Trauma Comfrey—the new improved cultivar—is even safer and more effective because it is free of potentially toxic PAs. So what can we expect from Trauma Comfrey botanicals grown and harvested under optimal conditions in Bavaria?

When we look at the solid body of research on Trauma Comfrey, we can see abundant evidence that, it does indeed have remarkable healing effects for sprains, strains, and bruises—and that the results hold true for children as well as adults. These effects are repeatedly documented:

1. Trauma Comfrey eases pain (that is, it is an anodyne).

2. Trauma Comfrey reduces inflammation and swelling (that is, it is anti-inflammatory).

3. Trauma Comfrey heals damage to soft tissue (that is, it is a cell proliferant).

By contrast, most topical gels or creams used in injuries are only analgesics that ease pain; a few are anti-inflammatories that reduce redness and swelling. None of them actually speed up the healing process itself by knitting soft tissue back together. Trauma Comfrey, on the other hand, has three powerful effects that are not duplicated anywhere. While Trauma Comfrey reduces pain, inflammation and swelling, it gets muscles, tendons and ligaments back into good working order. Unlike many NSAID-based or steroidal creams, it has virtually no side effects or interactions with any medications. It's so safe that it can even be used on children.

Let's look closer at some intriguing studies:

• A double-blind, randomized clinical trial studied 203 men and women in Prague between the ages of 18 and 50 who had sprained their ankles within the past 24 hours. Of those, 55% of the sprains occurred in sports, 29% at home, and 16% in a workplace. Half the participants were treated for 14 days with a Trauma Comfrey cream. The other half, the control group,

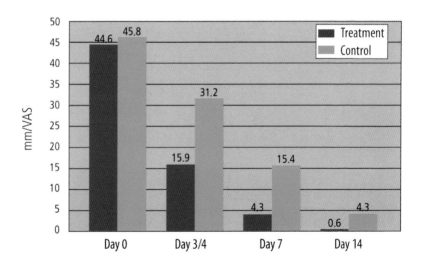

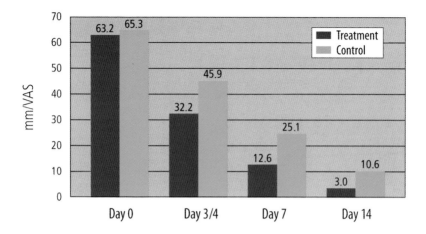

were treated with a salve that was indistinguishable by color, smell and texture from Trauma Comfrey plant but contained only a tenth as much of the active comfrey extract. The patients agreed to take no NSAIDs or do any kind of physiotherapy, but to massage two to three grams of the cream thoroughly into their ankles twice a day. The result: The sprained ankles in the Trauma Comfrey group improved more than *twice as fast* as the ankles of those taking the lower-dose placebo!

After three or four days of treatment, the participants were asked to walk 10 meters at a quick pace to assess their pain: the Trauma Comfrey patients reported the intensity of their pain had dropped by more than half, compared to a quarter in the control group. Careful measurements of the swelling showed a sharper reduction of three or four days with Trauma Comfrey. By Day 4, doctors reported that 85.6% of the Trauma Comfrey group showed good to excellent results, compared to 65.7 % of the control group. Age and gender made no difference—all patients responded well.

By the 14th and final day, 100 of the 103 Trauma Comfrey patients reported all the pain was gone! Only three patients with chronic conditions reported no improvement. Overall, doctors rated Trauma Comfrey as being "quick onset" or "very quick onset" of healing in 92 of the 103 patients. No adverse effects or drug interactions were reported.

- In another study, Trauma Comfrey was compared with conventional icepacks for treating patients with sprained ankles for two weeks. Not only did the patients do considerably better on the Trauma Comfrey, they were also more likely to rub on the cream than put on ice packs!

- Another study involved 14 men and eight women with "contusions and distortions of the knee joint"—bruised and sprained knees—who were treated with Trauma Comfrey 12 hours after getting injured, on average. They were told to rub the ointment into the wounded area at least four to five times a day—a relatively high dose—and then to bandage the wound and wrap it in gauze. The patients reported that when they put the ointment on, there was immediately a pleasant cooling sensation in the wounded area, followed by a distinct and prolonged drop in pain. Within four days, swelling and pain were markedly lowered. By day 7, none of the patients had pain while resting. Nineteen were completely pain-free even during movement by day 10 and the last three patients by day 14. No patient experienced any unpleasant reactions such as reddening, itching or drying out of the skin, and no systemic reactions in other parts of their bodies were observed. The study author noted that the quick drop in pain levels allowed the patients to move their knees sooner, diminishing the possibility of further muscle damage due to immobility.

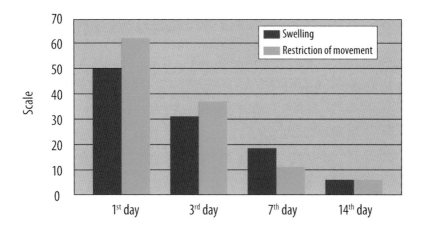

What about the children?

We're often worried about the effects of medicines on children, because their developing bodies make them vulnerable to too-potent doses and unforeseen side effects. But the scientific research on Trauma Comfrey holds only good news for them and their parents: It demonstrates that this powerful botanical quickly and effectively relieves pain and heals injuries without any negative effects.

• In a German study, 386 children between the ages of 3 and 12 who had suffered bruises, sprains, strains and muscle pain while playing sports were treated with Trauma Comfrey. It was judged 90% effective after two weeks of treatment. Importantly, the children tolerated Trauma Comfrey without any reactions or adverse effects.

• A total of 361 boys and girls between the ages of 4 and 12 who came to eight German clinics were treated with Trauma Comfrey for sprains, strains and bruises that had occurred in the previous 48 hours. Significant improvement for sprains occurred in just three days and in just four days for strains and bruises. Trauma Comfrey was found to be both safe and effective.

- In a third study, 196 children between 4 and 12 were treated with Trauma Comfrey for sprains, strains and bruises. Within eight days, pain while in motion and while being touched were both reduced an average of 86%, swelling was reduced 94%, and general impairment was reduced by 90%. No adverse drug reactions occurred.

What do these studies mean in practice?

If you or anyone you know gets a sprain, strain or bruise, hesitate not—reach for your tube of Trauma Comfrey! Even young children won't squirm when the non-greasy, non-stinging, slightly fragrant cream is rubbed on their skin. And you can breathe a little easier knowing that research fully supports you in doing your best in this way to heal the injury.

But what if the skin is broken? Open wounds and bad scrapes can be frightening to suffer and even look at, and in recent years, some people have hesitated to use comfrey on broken and bleeding skin. In the next chapter, we'll turn our attention to that discussion to see if Trauma Comfrey might play a role in those often-scary injuries.

CHAPTER FOUR

· · · · ·

Broken-Skin Wounds: Scrapes, Cuts, Punctures

Anyone who has ever learned to ride a bike—or who has helped a child learn—knows all about scraped knees. They come with the territory of growing up. They happen on playgrounds, baseball diamonds, soccer fields, on nature hikes, on rocks, around swimming pools—to children aged up to, oh, 80 or so!

Scraped knees or elbows—called "abrasions" by doctors—can look pretty frightening, especially if they're bleeding and encrusted with dirt. They're among the milder forms of what's known as "open wounds" or "broken-skin wounds," a category that also includes cuts and punctures.

Unlike sprains, strains and bruises, these injuries involve a break or tear in the skin and often produce bleeding. They're as common as, well, dirt! By the time we're adults, virtually everyone has scraped a knee, pricked a finger with a pin, or had a paper cut or worse. Thankfully, these are usually so mild that no medical care is necessary. Few statistics exist on them since there's no official government registry for scraped knees!

Even in sports, where scrapes and other wounds are an everyday matter, little hard information exists. As one sports-medicine researcher wrote in *The Journal of Athletic Training:* "Our impressions about wounds may be vivid, but our knowledge is vague.

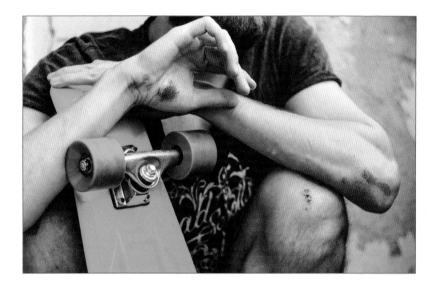

We do not know how frequently skin wounds occur, or how they occur. We do not even know individual characteristics about many wound types that might guide us in developing prevention strategies."

Nevertheless, there are enough sports wounds occurring that major U.S. hockey, baseball, basketball and soccer leagues enforce a written "blood rule" that requires an athlete with an open wound or bleeding to immediately leave the field to receive medical attention. (An interesting footnote: College soccer players suffer two to three times as many scrapes on artificial turf as on natural grass, according to one study.)

And indeed, there are some serious wounds, especially among kids, that merit trips to the emergency room. About two-thirds of the 12,000 Americans treated each day in hospital ERs for sports and recreation-incurred injuries are children aged 5 to 17. The great majority—98.7%—of them are treated and released as outpatients. Boys are three times as likely to be in the ER as girls.

The top five reasons are:

1. bruises

2. sprains and strains

3. arm fractures

4. open wounds of the head, neck and trunk

5. other injuries

Among the kids with open wounds, boys outnumbered girls five to one (22,300 to 4,300 patients). If you've got a boy, our sympathies!

It's important to treat open wounds quickly and effectively because by their very nature they carry risks of infection—indicated by tenderness, redness, oozing of smelly pus, red streaks or itching or boils around the wound. Infections can prove deadly and they're an outcome to avoid at all costs. With the serious nature of open wounds or punctures, always consult your physician before applying Trauma Comfrey.

Types of wounds

In general, open wounds are defined as injuries in which the skin is torn, cut or punctured. The most common ones include:

Abrasions (Scrapes)

These occur when skin comes into friction with something else, and they involve a scraping away of the top layer of skin (epidermis), often the layer of skin below that (dermis), and sometimes tissue and fat layers below the skin. Anytime we're moving fast and hit the ground—playing a hard game of tennis, roaring around in an ATV or motorbike, stumbling over a rock on a hike—we're prone to scrapes. Because nerve cells are exposed, abrasions can be very painful. They often need to be cleaned carefully to remove dirt and grit clinging to the wound surface.

Lacerations (Cuts)

These can have straight or jagged edges, and occur when the skin is penetrated or split open by an object. Employees who use sharp instruments and tools, especially kitchen and construction workers, are at high risk; even shaving every day is a bit of a risk! About 11 million cases occur annually in the U.S., with lacerations being the most common nonfatal injury among 10- to 17-year-olds.

Punctures

These are holes in the skin made by pointed objects—anything from paper edges and broken glass to knives, scissors, nails, sewing machine needles, farming tools, or building materials. They may penetrate body cavities and organs and are dangerous because of the possibility of infection if the edges of the wound close quickly before bacteria are neutralized. Because of this, check with your healthcare practitioner whenever you are in doubt about puncture wounds.

Two other types—penetration wounds, usually from knives or bullets, and pressure wounds, usually bedsores—can be life-threatening and go beyond home-based first aid to require immediate attention from a doctor.

How wounds are usually treated

For scrapes, cuts and punctures, treating wounds is a relatively straightforward process as the Mayo Clinic advises:

1. **Bleeding is stopped.** This is usually done by applying gentle, direct pressure with a clean cloth. The pressure is usually held continuously for about 10 to 20 minutes so that local blood vessels close off and blood is given time to clot. However, if the wound is likely to be contaminated, as in an animal bite or needle or other puncture injury, then bleeding is encouraged by squeezing the wound and running it under hot water to wash out bacteria and viruses.

2. **The wound is washed.** Plain old running water from a tap or salt water is best for this. To remove dirt and debris, the wound area can be gently scrubbed with a washcloth. Any foreign material in the wound, such as pebbles, grass or debris, can be removed gently by using fingers or tweezers. Hydrogen peroxide, Betadine (povidone-iodine), and detergents were once widely used to clean wounds, but their use has dropped because studies found they slowed wound healing in the long term. Even soap

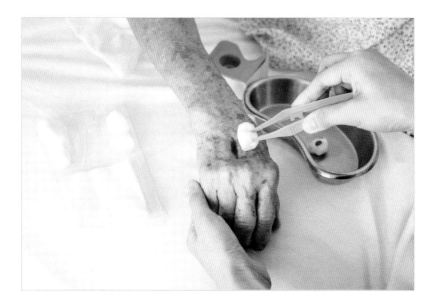

or detergents are no longer recommended by many experts because they can have toxic ingredients that interfere with healing, so plain water is best.

3. Skin may be rejoined. If the skin is not too damaged, the edges of the wound are put back together with certain types of bandages or tissue glue (liquid bandage). Deeper lacerations are stitched back together with sutures or staples, after the patient is given a local anesthesia. If the wound is deep enough to involve muscle, tendons and internal organs, emergency surgery may be required.

4. Ointment is applied. The wound is covered with ointment to keep the wound moist and prevent infection. In the United States, this is most often a first-aid antibiotic ointment such as Bacitracin, Neosporin or Polysporin. These, however, carry the possibility of an allergic reaction, especially Neosporin (neomycin), and that likelihood increases the more you use them. Even more seriously, a recent Japanese study in *Emerging Infectious Diseases* suggests that the overuse of antibiotic ointments may be contributing to the spread of antibiotic-resistant diseases like MRSA (methicillin-resistant *Staphylococcus aureus*), a disease responsible for an estimated 18,000 hospital deaths a year in the U.S. Trauma Comfrey is definitely a better choice, as we'll discuss later.

5. Bandages are applied. Wounds are typically wrapped with gauze or covered with a Band-Aid to help prevent infection and dirt from getting in the wound. If deemed necessary, the patient may be given a tetanus shot. If they've been exposed to human blood or bodily fluids, they may be immunized for hepatitis B or tested for HIV after an appropriate time period has passed.

If muscles and tendons have been hurt, rehabilitation exercises may be encouraged to prevent scar tissue from forming.

6. Follow-up. The wound should be washed, an ointment applied, and a bandage put over or around it three times a day.

You'll notice that comfrey is not a commonly used part of the above process—a most interesting fact, considering its documented history in healing open wounds.

Comfrey for wounds, past and present

Mention comfrey to an Emergency Room doctor, nurse or paramedic and you are likely to get a blank stare, at best. But if you had mentioned comfrey to a battlefield doctor in the armies of the Roman Empire, the Crusades, even the First World War, he might have handed you some comfrey ointment to start applying on the wounded men around you. For millennia, it was the best remedy for the ragged wounds of war.

As we touched on earlier, comfrey and other herbs fell out of favor in the 19th century, partly because scientists learned how to isolate certain active ingredients from herbs and synthesized them to develop pharmaceutical medicines, which were marketed as being "modern and quick-acting." Then, as these drugs' side-effects became apparent and interest revived in herbs in the late 20th century, scientists found that comfrey had certain constituents—PAs—that were toxic when fed to or injected into rats in large quantities. Although some countries consequently banned the use of comfrey in oral products such as teas, it was still permitted in skin salves because PAs have difficulty crossing the skin barrier. Still, many medical experts were concerned about that use and recommended that comfrey be used externally and only on closed-skin wounds for no more than 10 days.

The good news is that the concern is largely focused on comfrey root-based products, which can have a higher PA content than leaves, stems-and-flower-based preparations like those made from the Trauma Comfrey plant. And in fact, with Trauma Comfrey's total lack of PAs, prolonged use on broken skin no longer presents a danger—as emerging studies have repeatedly shown.

Comfrey does indeed have unique and powerful attributes to contribute to wound healing. In 1989, a German dermatologist and scientist named Dr. Roland Niedner became curious about comfrey's attributes and designed a study in which 10 healthy volunteers were pricked with needles to create three shallow wounds on their forearms. In each volunteer, two of the punctures were treated with the control substances—an oil and water ointment base on the first puncture, and a polyacrylamide agar gel on the second. The third puncture was treated with Trauma Comfrey

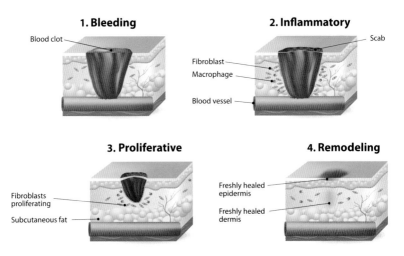

THE HEALING PROCESS

ointment. The results were dramatic: Trauma Comfrey healed the puncture wound in 3½ days—about two days sooner than the control substances, each of which was known to have some healing effects!

What created these remarkable results? Dr. Niedner pointed to:

- Allantoin, which helps create conditions in which new cells can grow rapidly to replace dying ones.

- Choline, which seals off capillaries and dilates blood vessels in the wound. This reduces the oozing of fluids out of inflamed tissues, draws infection-fighting white blood cells into the area, and helps to flush out metabolic wastes.

- Rosmarinic acid, which is anti-inflammatory, counters the oozing of fluid from cells and tissues, and slows down cell damage.

Dr. Niedner's pioneering study has been corroborated by recent rigorous studies that confirm the healing effects of Trauma Comfrey on open wounds—demonstrating that it dramatically hastens healing without side effects, even in that all-important group of children. Let's examine those studies.

What the research shows

One revealing study involved 189 people with fresh abrasions—63% of them got their scrapes during sports, 23% at home, 8% at work, and 6% in vehicles. Of those, 64 participants (23%) were children under age 20. One group was treated with a Trauma Comfrey cream; the other group was treated with a control cream that looked and felt identical to Trauma Comfrey but had a much lower potency, only a tenth of the comfrey extract.

In less than two days, the wounds in the Trauma Comfrey-treated patients shrunk by close to half—compared to a 25% shrinkage in the control group. That dramatic Trauma Comfrey effect took place at 1.4 days and wasn't reached by the control group until 2.4 days—a full day later. By the end of the study, the Trauma Comfrey group's wound healed in four days, compared to seven days for the control group—an impressive difference by any reckoning! Furthermore, doctors examining the patients rated the Trauma Comfrey as good or very good in 96% of the cases, compared to 61% in the control product.

In another rigorous study, a double-blind, randomized clinical trial, 108 children between 3 and 12 with fresh superficial skin abrasions were treated. None of them had been treated previously with antibiotic creams or topical disinfectants. About 41% of injuries occurred during sports, 39% in the home, 14% on the streets, 5% at school and % in leisure activities.

In half the cases, the child's wound was covered once a day with a thick layer of Trauma Comfrey and bandaged; in the other

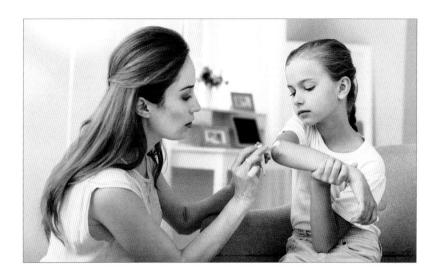

half of the cases, the child's wound was covered with a control product and was covered with a bandage. The outcome: Trauma Comfrey reduced the wound area to 50% approximately one day quicker than the control product did (1.8 vs. 2.7 days). Even the kids could tell the difference. They were asked to use "smileys" to show how effective they thought their cream was: 85% of the Trauma Comfrey kids rated it good or very good by the second or third day; the figure was 55% for the control product. No intolerance or skin irritations were seen in the youngsters.

And in another clinical trial that focused only on children, 326 youngsters from 3 to 15 years of age were treated who had mild abrasions or abrasions with associated bruising. After one week, Trauma Comfrey was rated 80% good or very good; after two weeks, the figure was 90%. No adverse events occurred—proving, once again, that Trauma Comfrey is safe and effective even for children.

What the studies mean in practice

Again, the broken-skin studies on Trauma Comfrey give us no cause to worry and much cause to celebrate. If you or your child scrape a knee while lunging for a softball, or get a small cut while slicing vegetables, you can wash the wound and then reach immediately for a tube of Trauma Comfrey. Studies show that its non-greasy, slightly fragrant cream, laden with the active ingredients of Trauma Comfrey, will soothe the pain immediately and go to work to repair the wound in record time. And worries about skin infection, allergic reactions or side effects need not cloud your mind during the recovery.

Trauma Comfrey is very good news for young, growing bodies—as well as for older bodies that get a few hard knocks. But the information about comfrey gets even better.

FUN FACTS ABOUT SKIN

- The skin is the largest organ in the body and contributes 12% to 15% of total body weight.

- The average human being has 21 square feet of skin and about 300 million skin cells.

- The skin is constantly renewing itself from the bottom up and takes 52 to 77 days to shed cells.

- By the age of 70, the average person will have lost 105 pounds of skin.

- Globally, dead skin accounts for about a billion tons of dust in the atmosphere. Your skin sheds 50,000 cells every minute.

- Each half-inch square of skin has approximately 10 hairs, 15 sebaceous glands, 100 sweat glands, and 3.2 feet of tiny blood vessels.

- White skin appeared just 20,000 to 50,000 years ago, as dark-skinned humans migrated to colder climates and lost much of their melanin pigment.

- Skin is thickest on the soles of the feet and thinnest on the eyelids.

- Skin emits up to 3 gallons of sweat per day.

- Skin expands in thickness from approximately 1 mm in babies to 2 mm in adults.

- Lip skin has a pigmented reddish tinge because it is very thin and the blood vessels show through.

Trauma Comfrey also produces impressive results for back pain, joint pain and muscle pain that can make life miserable on a minute-to-minute basis. Usually these are stubborn conditions that defy easy solutions—until now. Let's see what Trauma Comfrey can do to ease them.

CHAPTER FIVE

Soothing What Aches:
Back, Joint and Muscle Pain

"Oh, my aching back!"
"My knee really hurts!"
"It's painful to move—I must have pulled a muscle!"

It's the rare one among us who hasn't said each of these at least once in our life—sometimes all three on the same bad day! Activities such as playing racquetball too hard, gardening too vigorously, or sitting too long at the computer can bring on these aches and pains, particularly as we get up in years. In fact, more than half of American adults—215 million people—say they feel pain at one or more locations in their bodies at any given moment!

Although aches and pains can be part and parcel of more serious problems, most of the time they come and go. But if you're in the midst of a period of wrenching back or joint pain, it never goes away soon enough—indeed, does it ever go away soon enough?

Episodes of pain can last hours, days, weeks, months, even years. Even a brief one can wreak havoc on your home and work life. Lower back pain alone is the top reason that people under 45 cut back on their activities; it's the #2 reason people see their doctors and the #5 reason they go into hospitals. And for 20% of the population, pain is a chronic problem—with many depressing ramifications and few easy solutions.

Let's examine these painful conditions one by one, see what approaches exist to treat them, and then see how Trauma Comfrey can help return you to pain-free living.

Back pain

Back pain usually originates from the complex network of muscles, nerves, bones and joints that intersect in the spine. The pain may be constant or fluctuating, and it may be sharp, dull or piercing. It can stay in one place or spread to the arms and legs. Often back pain appears without any obvious cause. In fact, current practice among doctors is to treat the acute back pain first and worry about the diagnosis later.

How common is an aching back? Nine out of ten American adults will experience it in their lifetimes, and half of all working adults suffer it each year. Low back pain is the second most common cause of disability. Its costs are estimated between $100 and $200 billion annually in health care costs, decreased wages and

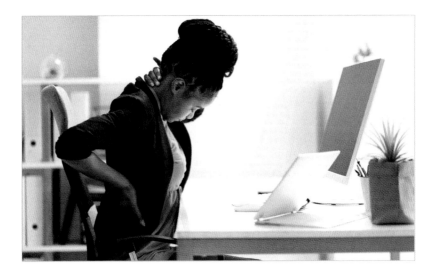

productivity. Back pain is second only to heart disease and cancer in its collective costs in medical care and disability payments, says the U.S. Agency for Healthcare Research and Quality. Treating back and neck problems costs about 10% of the entire costs of health care in the U.S. and leaps to about one-third of all health care costs when you roll in joint-related pain.

Some researchers call back pain an epidemic and point to such factors, including our relative inactivity compared to previous generations, hours spent sitting in front of screens of all kinds and the fact that two-thirds of us are overweight.

The good news is that 98% of back pain patients are diagnosed with "nonspecific acute back pain." That means there is not an underlying serious condition. About 80 to 90% of people with low back pain recover within six weeks and nearly 60% return to work within one week of the onset of pain. The bad news is that recurrences are common: 20-40% of workers report back pain returning within a year, and the lifetime recurrence rate is 85%.

If you have back pain, the impact on your life can be profound: Adults with low back pain are nearly three times as likely to report fair or poor health than those without back pain (26% vs. 9%), more than four times as likely to be unable to work, twice as likely to report less than six hours of sleep a night and seven times more likely to report psychological distress.

Who gets back pain? Just about everyone. It's common among children, the middle-aged, the elderly, manual workers, office workers, athletes and couch potatoes. It is more common among women than men, as well as for those living in a high-income country: Studies showed that people in Switzerland and Germany were three to four times more likely to have lower back pain than farmers toiling in the fields in Nigeria, China or Indonesia—but back pain is rising in those countries for factory and office workers.

Sometimes doctors can identify specific processes causing back pain, such as a pinched nerve, or a slipped disk, or irritation that causes inflammation in the muscles, bones, tendons or ligaments. But according to the National Pain Foundation, less than 15% of diagnosed back pain cases can be attributed to a particular cause.

Joint pain

The medical term for joint pain is *arthralgia*—from the Greek words for joint, *arthro* and pain, *algos*. The ancient Greeks suffered from arthralgia, as did the Romans, early Egyptians and Native Americans, as well as prehistoric peoples. Even dinosaurs, those rulers of the planet for eons, had ankle pain. Today in the United States, about 30% of adults report experiencing pain, aching or stiffness in a joint within the last 30 days—18% in the knee, 9% in the shoulder, 7% in the finger and 7%. As we get older, some of us may experience all of them at once!

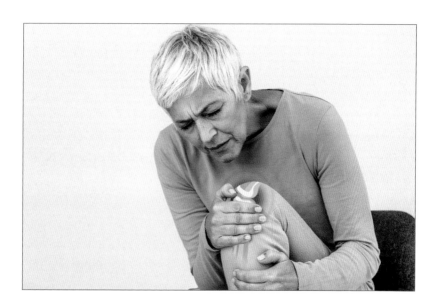

Joint pain—including aching, sharp pangs, swelling and stiffness can affect any part of your body, from your neck to your little toe. Injuries range from simple ones—like slamming a door on your finger or straining your shoulder while swinging a hammer—to life-numbing, chronic diseases like osteoarthritis, rheumatoid arthritis and lupus. It can be caused by injuries, infections, repetitive motions, conditions like gout or fibromyalgia, even medications. Advancing age makes joint pain more likely, as does being a woman.

Acute pain can last a few days or weeks or it can become chronic and last for months or years. If it is serious enough to hamper your activity, joint pain can make you much less active, contributing to weight gain, high cholesterol and heart disease. It tends to be worse in cold climates. If you're a long-distance runner, the high-impact activity makes knee pain more likely. If you sit in a chair all day at work, your knee joints also suffer.

Even if it's of short duration, joint pain tends to slow you down or even stop you in your tracks. If it lasts longer, it cramps your lifestyle. Adults with joint pain are 20 times more likely to report limiting their activities than joint-healthy people. They are four times as likely to be unable to work, twice as likely to sleep less than six hours a day and three times more likely to report being in distress psychologically, usually with depression. The annual cost in the U.S. is estimated to be $100 billion. Half of that is from people's lost earnings, so joint pain creates financial pain as well.

Muscle pain

The medical word for muscle pain—*myalgia*—also comes from the Greeks: *myo* means muscle, *algia* means pain. The body has 639 muscles and there might be times when you swear all of them hurt! Muscle pain can be a component of back or joint pain, or can occur when you overuse or injure a muscle (such as during sports) or when you're under tension (your tight shoulders after a tough day at work). It can hit when you get a sprain, strain, fracture or bruise. It can be caused by over-activity, if you push your body beyond its limits and also by under-activity, if you're a couch potato or have been sick. Did you ever notice how weak you feel after just a couple of days in bed with a cold?

Muscle pain can be a side effect of such popular drugs such as statins (one in 10 users report aching muscles), quino-lone antibiotics and SSRI and MAIO antidepressants. A simple electrolyte imbalance or vitamin D deficiency can cause muscle pain, but that pain can also be the major indicator of viruses like influenza, of infections like malaria and dengue 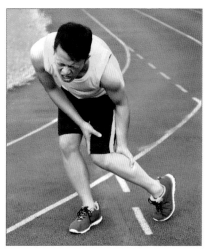 fever and of chronic illnesses like lupus and fibromyalgia.

Muscle pain can come on suddenly or slowly or it can be quite sharp and deep, accompanied by soreness, tenderness, difficulty moving the muscle and stiffness. It can be located by touch quite precisely on the body or it can involve a trigger point, a tender hardening in a muscle that evokes pain elsewhere in the body (called myofascial pain).

Muscle pain is very common: an estimated one in five people have chronic muscle pain, 1 in 50 has disabling fibromyalgia, and one in two elderly adults has nighttime muscle cramps, as do four in five pregnant women.

How back, joint and muscle pains are treated

There is a world of difference, of course, between a pulled shoulder muscle you got while swinging a golf club and a disabling condition of osteoarthritis that keeps you tied to the couch. Yet because back pain, joint pain and muscle pain all involve basic structures of bones, ligaments, tendons, fasciae and muscles, there are many common approaches to their treatments.

We'll look at those now, but first we must point out that both acute and chronic pain pose a real problem for doctors and all health professionals. There's no one-size-fits-all solution. Sometimes a diagnosis is obvious and helpful; more often the cause is a mystery and the prognosis and treatment uncertain. There are many studies on many treatments, but they often contradict each other. And every approach seems to have its own drawbacks. In the end, it too often falls upon you as the patient to sort through your options and try them out. The challenge is to persevere without losing heart, which I know is not easy when you're in pain.

Common approaches to treating and relieving pain include:

Medications

Non-steroidal anti-inflammatory drugs (NSAIDs), both over-the-counter and prescription, are typically given for pain. NSAIDs such as aspirin, ibuprofen (Motrin) and naproxen (Aleve) are usually better at relieving pain than acetaminophen (Tylenol), studies show. The drawbacks of NSAIDs, however, are substantial: They can cause serious toxicity problems and gastric bleeding resulting in hospitalization for as many as 200,000 Americans each year, killing over 17,000 people annually. NSAID use can double your risk of heart attack and stroke because the drugs decrease kidney function. Acetaminophen overdose—usually accidental, because it is included in so many meds and interacts with alcohol—is the leading cause of acute liver failure in developed countries, and accounts for 26,000 hospitalizations and 500 deaths a year in the U.S.

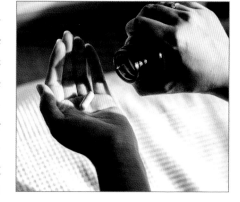

Depending on the diagnosis, doctors may prescribe other medications, such as narcotic painkillers, muscle relaxants, immunosuppressants or antibiotics. They may take you off medications that sometimes bring on joint pain, such as statins for cholesterol, proton pump inhibitors for gastroesophageal reflux disease (GERD) or bisphosphonates for osteoporosis. We all have heard of the terrible opioid epidemic, which is driven large by the demand for pain relief that ends all too often in addiction.

Surgery

For an aching back, surgery is considered the remedy of last resort. Fewer than 10%—some say just 1%—of back pain cases

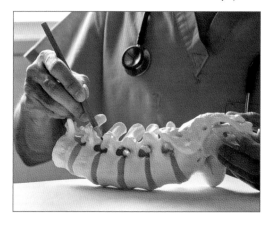

are caused by the rare conditions that merit such an invasive procedure, and its benefits decline in the long term. Back surgery has sometimes been called sham surgery because it has such a high failure rate.

Knee replacement surgery is another story: those operations are up 162% in the past two decades, according to the *Journal of the American Medical Association*. Knee and hip replacement have relieved pain and restored mobility for millions of aging Americans, with a success rate of about 90%. The drawbacks are that it is major surgery, which means it is costly, can have complications and involves physical therapy and a long recovery. And as our longevity continues to increase, there is the chance that the procedure will need to be repeated in a few decades.

Injections

For stubborn joint pain, especially in the knee or shoulder, doctors may inject a steroid medication or hyaluronan, which mimics joint fluid, into the joint every three or four months. The drawback is that both types of injections have temporary effects and they may become less effective with repeated treatments. Some studies find injections ineffective and they can cause such side effects as bruising, infection, tendon weakening 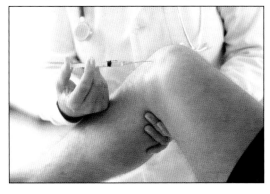 and nerve damage. There are also suggestions that the corticosteroids migrate to surrounding body tissues and bone increasing the risk of weakening joints, osteoporosis and fractures. Common side effects of steroid injections include increased blood pressure, increased blood sugar, loss of potassium, immune system suppression, anxiety, insomnia, fluid retention, headache, mood swings and muscle weakness.

Spine adjustments

Osteopathic physicians and chiropractors, who are intensively trained in the management of musculoskeletal disorders, treat back, joint and muscle pain by moving joints back into place, massaging soft tissue and helping stressed muscles to relax. A recent study found that osteopathy reduced chronic back pain better than a sham treatment or electrotherapy. And another study found that more than twice as many people with neck pain became pain-free with chiropractic as opposed to

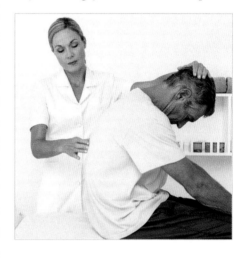

medication. The drawback is that it can take time for treatments to take effect and you'll have to seek a good practitioner, plus paying for it may not be covered by insurance, so it can be an out-of-pocket expense that can mount up quickly.

Physical therapy

Stretching exercises and gentle routines that strengthen the core and posture of the body are frequently taught by physical therapists in hospitals, rehab clinics and health spas. Studies show that the right exercises can ease pain, improve function and decrease the need for surgery, especially among those of us who sit in front of screens all day. Therapists also show you how to avoid future pain by using an ergonomic chair and keeping your computer screen at eye level, by using lumbar support for the hollow of your back and by leaning the proper way to lift heavy objects. The drawback? Therapy takes time, effort and work.

Stress relief

Emotions such as fear, anger and grief, especially if they are suppressed, can play a role in physical pain, studies have shown. Cognitive therapy and brief trauma therapy such as EMDR (eye movement desensitization and reprocessing) can help, as does the educational approach pioneered by John Sarno, M.D., of New York University, who says pain often stems from buried emotional issues that trigger tension in the body and ultimately deprive nerves and muscles of oxygen. The drawback is that it is challenging to address deeper emotional issues because, well, they hurt!

Heat therapy

Conventional wisdom says to cool a recent injury, applying ice packs for 20 minutes every hour for the first three days.

One study found that heat works for many patients with sudden back pain—either moist heat (as in a hot bath) or continuous heat, such as a heat wrap that stays warm from four to six hours.

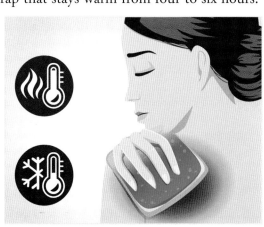

Other patients report that cold—a pack of ice or frozen vegetables wrapped in a towel—helps them.

One common recommendation is to alternate between heat and cold, with

15 minutes of heat, 15 minutes of cold, 30 minutes of neither, then start the cycle over again.

Acupuncture, acupressure and massage

Some back-pain sufferers swear by these. A *Consumers Report* subscriber survey found that for back pain, 51% of people say that deep-tissue massage "helped a lot," 45% said the same of acupressure and 41% of acupuncture. A review by the well-respected Cochrane Collaboration found long-term benefit for low back pain from acupressure, and said it seemed more effective than Swedish massage. The drawbacks? Again, finding a good practitioner and paying for the services, which are rarely covered by insurance.

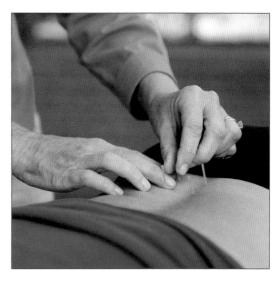

Supplements

People in pain have found relief from a number of herbs, vitamins and other supplements, many of which are well-researched and have proven their value over time. There is an exhaustive list of potential supplement interventions, but some of the best are curcumin, boswellia, ginger and omega-3 fatty acids (EPA and DHA).

We personally recommend curcumin and boswellia without reservation, for long-term pain and even for quick relief for a sudden onset of pain. There is a large amount of research on curcumin's effectiveness for joint pain as well as a variety of other conditions. For instance, one human study on rheumatoid arthritis found that a form called BCM-95 curcumin is much better absorbed by the body and provides the same amount of pain relief and improved mobility as the popular but risky prescription drug diclofenac sodium (Voltaren). For more information, you can read about curcumin's extensive healing effects in Dr. Jan McBarron's book *Curcumin: The 21st Century Cure.*

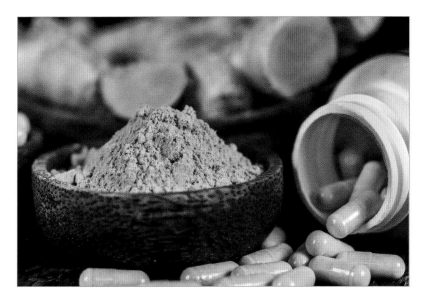

Salves, ointments, creams

Rubbing a pain-relieving cream on a sore or aching spot is perhaps the easiest, most pleasant therapy for pain. There are three popular types of topical agents:

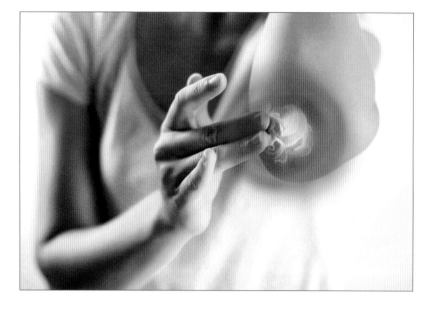

1. **BENGAY and friends.** Menthol, camphor and methylsalicylate products create a burning or cooling sensation that distracts your mind from pain. Side effects can include skin rash and irritation and, if used in huge quantities, nausea and ringing in the ears.

2. **Hot chili peppers.** Capsaicin creams cause a warm tingling sensation that helps block pain signals and triggers the release of relaxing endorphins. The drawback is that it sometimes burns too much and it can take several weeks for results to kick in.

3. **Topical non-steroidal anti-inflammatory drugs (NSAIDs).** In Europe, NSAIDs in the form of topical creams are the preferred form for treating hand and knee osteoarthritis and rheumatism, and in the last few years, topical NSAIDs have been appearing in the US, to much excitement. They have been found to be as effective as NSAIDs pills in treating conditions like muscle

soreness and tendonitis, and because they bypass the stomach, appear to have fewer side effects such as indigestion, diarrhea, abdominal pain, liver damage and anemia. The drawbacks: Redness, irritation, dry skin and rash are still common, and the three topical NSAIDs sold in the US all contain diclofenac, whose oral version is linked to liver damage.

Now, look closely. What's missing from this list of approaches that heal pain?

Right! Comfrey!

Read on. We'll be filling you in on all the details, explaining why Trauma Comfrey is the right stuff, the safe stuff and the healing cream you want.

CHAPTER SIX

Know How to Make the Right Choice

EXPERT ADVICE FROM TERRY LEMEROND

I've been researching and studying a broad range of nutritional supplements and botanicals for over 50 years. It is my passion and my life's work. I love the fact that we can recommend the humble comfrey plant which has been used as a medicinal for millennia in a way that is safe and effective by today's terms. That's amazing news!

I'm sure you're convinced by the preponderance of this evidence that Trauma Comfrey is the plant you need to heal those sprains, strains, stings, bites, and pains of everyday life.

As you've read, our ancestors have been using this special cultivar of the comfrey plant for thousands of years. They spent a great deal of time preparing a natural, healing cream that provided the relief they needed.

You'll be glad to learn that as modern-day-science validates the healing power of Trauma Comfrey, there is now a product that can save you all the mess and bother. All you have to do is squeeze a lightly scented creme from a tube several times a day and voila! Healing.

You'll remember that the allantoin component of the Trauma Comfrey plant is a key ingredient.

First, be sure you have a product with the correct cultivar, Trauma Comfrey (*Symphytum x uplandicum NYMAN*). That is the only cultivar that is free of toxic pyrrolizidine alkaloids (PAs) that can cause liver problems if taken internally in high doses. Of course, you won't be taking it internally at all and the absorption through the skin, even if you use it several times a day, won't be a problem but why take any risk when we have such a perfect variety available? That's why Trauma Comfrey is so important.

Trauma Comfrey products are made from the leaves and stems of the plant, not the roots, which can have high concentration of

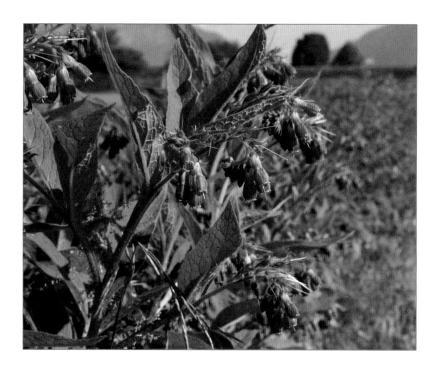

PAs. The aerial plant parts are rich in the key healing components of Trauma Comfrey: rosmarinic acid, allantoin and choline. You'll want a product the verifies it contains at least 10% of these crucial ingredients.

To ensure safety, look for a product produced without chemical pesticides or artificial fertilizers, with aqueous extraction (rather than some that might use toxic chemical solvents) and is free of hormone-disrupting parabens that are often used in as preservatives in cosmetics and first aid creams.

Sixteen European studies confirm that Trauma Comfrey is effective in relieving pain, speeding healing and all without side effects.

What the research shows about Trauma Comfrey and pain relief

As it turns out, the research on Trauma Comfrey will give you reason to smile through your pain.

And, unlike the approaches to pain we've just been discussing, *there are virtually no drawbacks in terms of time, expense, effort or side effects.* That's a huge recommendation in itself.

Trauma Comfrey can dramatically slash muscle pain in a wide range of conditions, one study found Trauma Comfrey was 90 to 100% effective within 14 days in removing all pain and movement problems. It has surprisingly strong effect on stubborn conditions like degenerative joint pain, vertebral syndrome and enthesopathy (disorders affecting ligaments and tendons and how they attach to bone), with an improvement rate of 75% or more.

Back pain, too, can be knocked back with Trauma Comfrey, as verified by another study. The doctors in the Czech Republic who did the previous study—professors in the Department of Sports

Medicine and Rehabilitation at Charles University in Prague, Czech Republic—found that people with long-term back pain problems reported that their pain had dropped by 90% in the Trauma Comfrey group, but by only 50% for the control group.

What the studies mean for you

The research resoundingly demonstrates that whether you suffer an occasional injury or bout of pain or live with it on a daily basis, Trauma Comfrey can help you. Its robust active ingredients—allantoin, choline and rosmarinic acid—effectively penetrate the skin to provide deep relief for pain, aches, injuries, stiffness, and swelling. It can easily be used alone, to soothe an aching back after a hard day at a computer, to massage into a shoulder or leg after a hard-played softball game, or to soothe aching, aging fingers.

It can also be used along with mainstream approaches like rehabilitation exercises and frozen-shoulder treatments without any contraindications.

And because it's free of side effects and reactions with medications, it can't hurt to combine it with such approaches as acupressure, spinal adjustments or supplements, even during recovery from surgery.

How often should you use Trauma Comfrey? Whenever you want! Three times a day was the amount used in most studies, but because of its high safety profile, there are no cautions about the amount or frequency of use.

You can easily buy Trauma Comfrey online or at quality health food store and at integrative medical offices. I recommend that you keep it on hand for those pitfalls of daily life.

CHAPTER SEVEN

· · · · ·

From the Doctor

Dear Readers,
This chapter is written for your doctor or health care practitioner. We all realize that our health care experts are very busy and unlikely to be able to carve out the time to read this entire book. That is why we urge you to copy this synopsis of the science behind Trauma Comfrey and hand it to your doctor.

From Dr. Lucille:

Like most books, this book is copyrighted. However, the information presented here is so important to your patients' health and to your scientific knowledge that we have urged our readers to copy this chapter and give it to you in hope that this brief summary of efficacy of *Symphytum x uplandicum NYMAN*, commonly known as Trauma Comfrey, to treat wounds and chronic pain situations safely and effectively.

I appreciate the time you've devoted to this material. I promise it will be brief!

First, let me introduce myself:

I am Holly Lucille, ND, RN. My professional degrees in conventional and holistic medicine are a combination that I think give me a unique integrative perspective on health and healing. It is from this viewpoint I ask you to consider Trauma Comfrey as a safe and efficacious treatment for wounds, joint pain and soft tissue injuries. I have recommended it to my patients and my colleagues for years. Now I hope to spread the message even farther.

"Wait!" you might be thinking. "Comfrey is toxic."

Yes, comfrey, taken internally has had some toxic effects. Even some topical applications have shown adverse effects. The Trauma Comfrey healing cream I recommend comes from the leaves and stems of the cultivar *Symphytum x uplandicum NYMAN,* which are completely free of a pyrrolizidine alkaloids, that may be hepatotoxic especially when in internally by patients who are liver compromised or are taking certain pharmaceuticals. There's no need for concern with products made from this cultivar. It is also aqueous processed to avoid the introduction of solvents as is found in many inexpensive products.

The Trauma Comfrey cultivar has been empirically confirmed with the following properties:

Anti-bacterial	Kills or slows down growth of bacteria
Anti-exudative	Counters the oozing of fluid from cells and tissues as a result of inflammation or injury
Anti-fungal	Fights fungus invaders such as yeast, mold and rot
Anti-inflammatory	Prevents or reduces inflammation in cells
Anodyne	Relieves pain
Antiseptic	Kills or retards the growth of infection-causing microorganisms
Demulcent	Soothes pain in inflamed tissues, especially mucous membranes
Emollient	Softens the skin
Styptic	Arrests bleeding by contracting blood vessels
Vulnerary	Heals fresh wounds

Here is a brief laundry list of the study-validated benefits of using a Trauma Comfrey cream:

- Heals sprained ankles in half the time of those treated with placebo.

- Reduces pain and immobility in injured knees by 75% in just seven days.

- Shaves three days off full recovery from abrasions.

- Shrinks abrasions in adults and children in half the time compared to placebo.

- Reduces by at least three days rehabilitation for a frozen shoulder.

- Cuts the immobility of acute back pain by 66% within three days.

- Relieves pain by 90 to 100% in locomotor problems with strong muscular components, and can even ease pain in some degenerative conditions.

- Is so safe that it accelerates the healing process for children as young as four without any reactions or adverse effects.

We now know that the constituents in comfrey, especially allantoin, choline and rosmarinic acid, are the active ingredients as anti-inflammatories, assisting in wound remodeling and stimulating cell proliferation. Even as pain is eased, damaged skin, tendons, cartilage, fasciae and bones are quickly repaired.

In study after study, absolutely no interactions were found between Trauma Comfrey and other medications or supplements. No systemic effects were found on other organs, and no side effects were experienced, with one small exception: In less than 1% of cases, some slight reddening of the skin occurred where the ointment was applied, apparently due to a rare allergic reaction to its non-comfrey part. The irritation typically faded without further treatment.

Trauma Comfrey cream has been proven to be safe and highly effective, opening up new horizons for trauma-care doctors. I wish you and your patients healing and health with Trauma Comfrey.

References

Chapter One

Grieve, M. *Comfrey, A Modern Herbal.* Dover Publications, New York, 1971. http://botanical.com/botanical/mgmh/c/comfre92.html.

MacAlister, CJ, Titherley AW. *Narrative of an Investigation Concerning an Ancient Medicinal Remedy and its Modern Utilities Together with an Account of the Chemical Constitution of Allantoin.* John Bale, Sons, and Danielsson. 1936.

Teynor TM, Putnam DH, et al. "Comfrey," Alternative Field Crops Manual. University of Wisconsin, Division of Cooperative Extension of UWEX, Madison, Wis. 2013. http://corn.agronomy.wisc.edu/Crops/Comfrey.aspx

Chapter Two

Hirono I, Haga M, Fujii M, et al. Induction of hepatic tumors in rats by senkirkine and symphytine. *J Natl Cancer Inst.* 1979;63(2):469–472.

Schmidt M, High-performance cultivar 'Harras' as a contribution to quality, efficacy and safety of comfrey. *Journal of Medicinal & Spice Plants.* 2008 Dec; 13: 182–184.

Stickel F, Seitz HK. The efficacy and safety of comfrey. *Public Health Nutr.* 2000;3:501–8

Weston CF, Cooper BT, Davies JD, Levine DF. Veno-occlusive disease of the liver secondary to ingestion of comfrey. *Br Med J (Clin Res Ed).* 1987 Jul 18; 295(6591):183.

Yeong ML, Swinburn B, Kennedy M, Nicholson G. Hepatic veno-occlusive disease associated with comfrey ingestion. *Gastroenterol Hepatol.* 1990 Mar–Apr; 5(2):211–4.

Chapter Three

Adirim TA, Cheng TL. Overview of injuries in the young athlete. *Sports Med.* 2003;33:75–81.

Hess H. Effect of a Symphytum Ointment with Sports Injuries of the Knee Joint. *German J Sports Med.* 1991;42:156–162.

Requa RK, DeAvilla LN, Garrick JG. Injuries in recreational adult fitness activities. *Am J Sports Med.* 1993 May–Jun;21(3):461–467.

Kucera M, Barna M, Horacek O, et al. Efficacy and safety of topically applied *Symphytum* herb extract cream in the treatment of ankle distortion: results of a randomized controlled clinical double blind study. *Wien Med-Wochenschr.* 2004;154:498–507

Marshall SW, Guskiewicz KM. Sports and recreational injury: the hidden cost of a healthy lifestyle. *Inj Prev.* 2003; 9:100–102.

Mayer G. The Local Treatment of Acute Lateral Distortions of the Ankle Joint with an Ointment Containing Symphytum Active Substance Complex. *Acta Therapeutica.* 1991 April; 17:89–100.

Mayer G. The Local Treatment of Contusions and Distortions of the Knee Joint with a Symphytum Active Substance Complex Ointment. *Erfahrungsheilkunde.* 1992;12:888–891.

Moore RA, Tramer MR, et al. Quantitative systematic review of topically applied non-steroidal anti-inflammatory drugs. *Br Med J.* 1998; 316:333–338

Rutherford GJ, Schroeder T. Sports-related Injuries to Persons 65 Years of Age and Older. Washington, DC: US Consumer Products Safety Commission; 1998:4.

Staiger C. Comfrey: A Clinical Overview. *Phytother Res.* 2012 Oct: 1441–48.

Travisano D. What you don't know about sports injuries can really hurt you. *Sports Injury Bul,* http://www.sportsinjurybulletin.com/archive/0123a-sport-injuries.htm.

Chapter Four

Author unknown. "The Skin You're In—Fun Facts." Association for the Advancement of Wound Care. http://aawconline.org/the-skin-you percentE2 percent80 percent99re-in-fun-facts/

Barna M, Kucera A, et al, Randomized Double-Blind Study: Wound-Healing Effects of a Symphytum Herb Extract Cream in Children. *Arzneimittelforschung Drug Research.* 2012; 62:285–289.

Barna M, Kucera A, Hladicova M, et al. Wound healing effects of a Symphytum herb extract cream (Symphytum x uplandicum NYMAN): Results of a randomized, controlled double-blind study. *Wien Med Wochenschr.* 2007;157:569–574.

Forsch, RT, Essentials of Skin Laceration Repair. *Am Fam Physician.* 2008 Oct 15;78(8):945-951.

Foster DT, Rowedder LJ, Reese SK. Management of Sports-Induced Skin Wounds. *J of Athl Training.* 1995:30:135–139.

Niedner R., Effect of an Active Substance Complex from Symphytum on Epithelialization. *Acta Therapeutica.* 1989; 15:289–297.

Wier L, Miller A., Steiner, C., Sports Injuries in Children Requiring Hospital Emergency Care, 2006. HCUP Statistical Brief #75. June 2009. Agency for Healthcare Research and Quality, Rockville, MD

Chapter Five

Author unknown. "Alternative treatments: More than 45,000 readers tell us what helped." Consumer Reports Online. July 2011. http://www.consumerreports.org/cro/2012/04/alternative-treatments/index.htm

Freburger JK, Holmes GM, et al, The Rising Prevalence of Chronic Low Back Pain. *Arch Intern Med.* 2009;169(3):251–258.

Guth A, Mercekova L et al. Final Report of the Monitoring of the Rehabilitation in Cervical Spine Functional Disorders in Medication Coverage with the Help of Trauma Comfrey. *Aertz Rundschau,* 2009.

Jorge LL, Feres CC, et al. Topical preparations for pain relief: efficacy and patient adherence. *J Pain Res.* 2011; 4:11–24.

Kucera M, Kalal J, Polesna Z. Effects of Symphytum ointment on muscular symptoms and functional locomotor disturbances. *Adv Ther.* 2000;17:204–210.

Kucera M, Barna M, et al. Topical Symphytum Herb Concentrate Cream against Myalgia. *Adv Ther.* 2005;22:681–692

Martin, B, Deyo, RA, et. al. Original Contribution Expenditures and Health Status Among Adults With Back and Neck Problems. *JAMA.* 2008;299(6):656–664.

Mayer G. The Local Treatment of Acute Supraspinatus Tendon Syndrome with a Symphytum Active Substance Complex Ointment. *German J Sports Med.* 1993;44:121–124.

Paulose R, Hertz RP. *The burden of pain among adults in the United States.* Pfizer Medical Division, 2008. 93pp.

Soni, A. *Back Problems: Use and Expenditures for the U.S. Adult Populations, 2007.* Statistical Brief #289. Medical Expenditure Panel Survey. Agency for Healthcare Research and Quality. 2010 July.

Suzuki, M. et al. Antimicrobial Ointments and Methicillin-Resistant Staphylococcus aureus USA300, *Emerging Infectious Diseases.* 2011 October; 15:1,19–23.

Tarkan L. "Topical gel catches up with pills for relief." *New York Times,* Sept. 6, 2010. http://www.nytimes.com/2010/09/07/health/07pain.html

Violinn E., The epidemiology of low back pain in the rest of the world. *Spine.* 1997 Aug 1;22(15):1747–54.

Index

About the Authors

DR. HOLLY LUCILLE

Dr. Holly Lucille, a.k.a. "Dr. Holly," is a nationally recognized and licensed practicing naturopathic doctor, natural products consultant and television & radio host.

An acclaimed expert in the field of integrative medicine, Dr. Holly lectures throughout the nation on a variety of natural health topics. Her appearances include national media programs and networks including *Dr. Oz, The Doctors, Lifetime Television for Women, Montel Williams, PBS's Healing Quest, The Hallmark Channel* and *Discovery Fit & Health Channel.* She is on the editorial advisory board of Alternative Medicine and Natural Practitioner and is also regularly quoted as an expert in both consumer and peer journals. In 2007, Dr. Holly was listed in *Time Magazine*'s "Alt List" as one of the "Top 100 Most Influential People." In 2012 she launched her own talk show, "Myth-Defying with Dr. Holly," on the Veria Living Network and is the co-host of "It's Your Health & It Ain't Rocket Science" radio show on RadioMD.

Dr. Holly believes in the science, art and mystery of healing and has a heartfelt passion for the individual wellness of all people. Built on this foundational belief, Dr. Holly's private practice in Los Angeles, Healing from Within Healthcare, focuses on comprehensive naturopathic medicine and individualized care.

Dr. Holly is the past president of the California Naturopathic Doctors Association where she worked to ensure the availability of safe naturopathic health care by spearheading a lobbying effort to have naturopathic doctors licensed in the state of California. She has also worked with the LA Free Clinic providing health education, promotion and prevention in the public health system and recently was awarded the "SCNM Legacy Award" for her "contribution to the advancement and development of the field of naturopathic medicine." Dr. Holly graduated from the Southwest College of Naturopathic Medicine in Tempe, AZ where she received the prestigious Daphne Blayden Award for her "commitment to naturopathic medicine, academic excellence, compassion, perseverance, a loving sense of humor and a positive, supportive outlook."

Also known as the "Daredevil Doctor," Dr. Holly enjoys riding motorcycles, competing in Crossfit competitions and going off the beaten path in nature.

Find her at: drhollylucille.com

TERRY LEMEROND

Terry Lemerond is a natural health expert with over 50 years of experience helping people live healthier, happier lives. A much sought-after speaker and accomplished author, Terry shares his wealth of experience and knowledge in health and nutrition through his educational programs, including the *Terry Talks Nutrition* website—TerryTalksNutrition.com—newsletters, podcasts, webinars, and personal speaking engagements. Terry has also hosted *Terry Talks Nutrition radio* for the past 30 years. His books include *Seven Keys to Vibrant Health, Seven Keys to Unlimited*

Personal Achievement, and *50+ Natural Health Secrets Proven to Change Your Life.* Terry continues to author and co-author books to educate everyone on the steps they can take to live a more healthy, vibrant life.

His continual dedication, energy, and zeal are part of his ongoing mission—to help us all improve our health.

KNOWLEDGE IS POWER,
ESPECIALLY FOR YOUR HEALTH!

Are you in search of a reliable, science-based resource for all your health and nutrition questions? Terry Talks Nutrition has you covered.

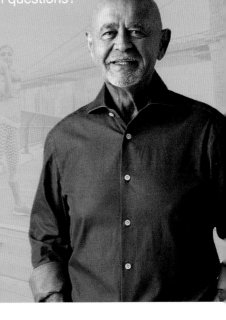

Connect with Terry to increase your knowledge on a wide variety of topics, including immunity, pain, curcumin and cancer, diabetes, and so much more!

READ

Visit TerryTalksNutrition.com for today's latest and greatest health and nutrition information.

LISTEN

Tune in on Sat. and Sun. 8-9 am (CST) at TerryTalksNutrition.com for a live internet radio show hosted by Terry! You can listen to past shows on the website or on your favorite podcast app.

ENGAGE

Connect with us on Facebook, where you can engage with other individuals seeking safe and effective ways to improve overall wellness.

WATCH

Check out our educational YouTube Channel to learn from the world's leading doctors and health experts.

Simply open your smartphone camera. Hold over desired code above for more information.

Get answers to all of your health questions at **TERRYTALKSNUTRITION.COM**

WELCOME TO

ttn
publishing

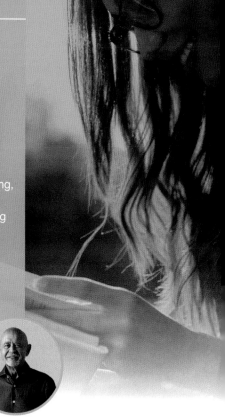

Are you ready to learn how anyone can use natural medicines, safely and effectively, to improve their health? You'll love TTN Publishing, my newest endeavor to bring you cutting edge research on powerful, health-supporting botanicals. I've coauthored numerous books with top alternative doctors from around the world to help you learn all you can about taking your health into your own hands. These educational books, supported by powerful scientific research, contain all the information you need to live a life of vibrant health.

In Good Health,
Terry Lemerond

BROUGHT TO YOU BY TTN PUBLISHING:

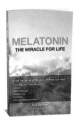
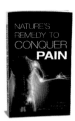
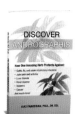
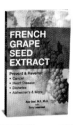

Get a copy for yourself and gift them to the people you care about!

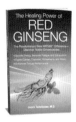
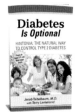
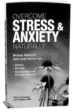
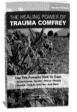
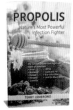

Available at your local health food store or online.

Visit TTNPublishing.com for more news and our latest publications.

TTNPUBLISHING.COM | info@ttnpublishing.com